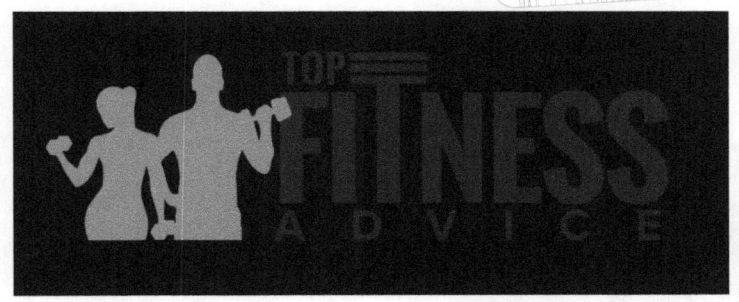

STRESS

3ᵈ Edition

17 Stress Management Habits to Reduce Stress, Live Stress-Free & Worry Less!

LINDA WESTWOOD

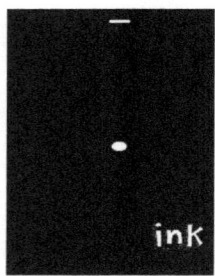

First published in 2015 by Venture Ink Publishing

Copyright © Top Fitness Advice 2019

All rights reserved.

No part of this book may be reproduced in any form without permission in writing from the author. No part of this publication may be reproduced or transmitted in any form or by any means, mechanic, electronic, photocopying, recording, by any storage or retrieval system, or transmitted by email without the permission in writing from the author and publisher.

Requests to the publisher for permission should be addressed to publishing@ventureink.co

For more information about the contents of this book or questions to the author, please contact Linda Westwood at linda@topfitnessadvice.com

Disclaimer

This book provides wellness management information in an informative and educational manner only, with information that is general in nature and that is not specific to you, the reader. The contents of this book are intended to assist you and other readers in your personal wellness efforts. Consult your physician regarding the applicability of any information provided in this book to you.

Nothing in this book should be construed as personal advice or diagnosis, and must not be used in this manner. The information provided about conditions is general in nature. This information does not cover all possible uses, actions, precautions, side-effects, or interactions of medicines, or medical procedures. The information in this book should not be considered as complete and does not cover all diseases, ailments, physical conditions, or their treatment.

You should consult with your physician before beginning any exercise, weight loss, or health care program. This book should not be used in place of a call or visit to a competent health-care professional. You should consult a health care professional before adopting any of the suggestions in this book or before drawing inferences from it.

Any decision regarding treatment and medication for your condition should be made with the advice and consultation of a qualified health care professional. If you have, or suspect you have, a health-care problem, then you should immediately contact a qualified health care professional for treatment.

No Warranties: The author and publisher don't guarantee or warrant the quality, accuracy, completeness, timeliness, appropriateness or suitability of the information in this book, or of any product or services referenced in this book.

The information in this book is provided on an "as is" basis and the author and publisher make no representations or warranties of any kind with respect to this information. This book may contain inaccuracies, typographical errors, or other errors.

Liability Disclaimer: The publisher, author, and other parties involved in the creation, production, provision of information, or delivery of this book specifically disclaim any responsibility, and shall not be held liable for any damages, claims, injuries, losses, liabilities, costs, or obligations including any direct, indirect, special, incidental, or consequences damages (collectively known as "Damages") whatsoever and howsoever caused, arising out of, or in connection with the use or misuse of the site and the information contained within it, whether such Damages arise in contract, tort, negligence, equity, statute law, or by way of other legal theory.

Table of Contents

Disclaimer	3
Who is this book for?	9
What will this book teach you?	11
Introduction	13
Stress Buster 1: Stop the Caffeine Binge	19
Stress Buster 2: Take Control of the Controllable	27
Stress Buster 3: Emotional Eating the RIGHT Way	33
Stress Buster 4: The ONE HABIT That WILL Extend Your Life	39
Stress Buster 5: You Could Already Be Doing This WRONG	45
Stress Buster 6: Rest Your Mind Regularly	51
Stress Buster 7: Rest Your Body Regularly	57
Stress Buster 8: Read Every Day	63
Stress Buster 9: Shift Negative Hobbies	69
Stress Buster 10: Be Realistic About Time	75
Stress Buster 11: Let Others Help You!	81
Stress Buster 12: Hang Out with Family & Friends	87

Stress Buster 13: Get Things Done NOW   93

Stress Buster 14: Alter Your Mind   97

Stress Buster 15: Slow Down   103

Stress Buster 16: I Don't Care   109

Stress Buster 17: Limit Your Chemical Intake   113

Conclusion   121

Final Words   127

Would you prefer to listen to my book, rather than read it?

Download the audiobook version for free!

If you go to the special link below and sign up to Audible as a new customer, you can get the audiobook version of my book completely free.

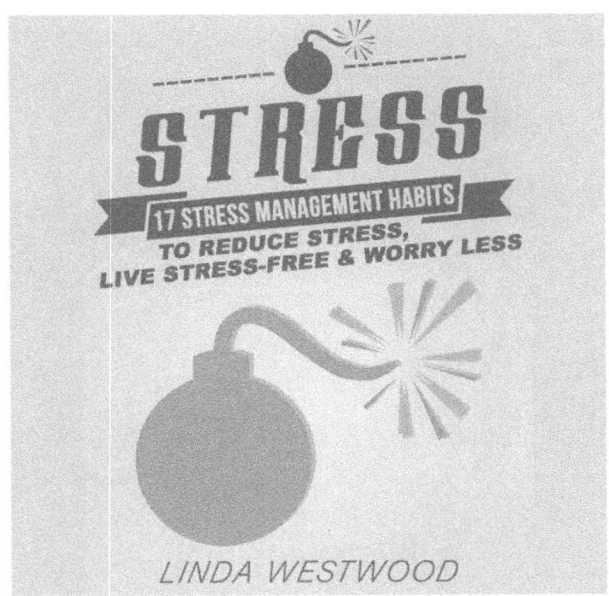

Go here to get your audiobook version for free:

TopFitnessAdvice.com/go/stress

Who is this book for?

Do you feel like stress sometimes just overwhelms you?

Are you struggling with feeling pressured, anxious or even stressed?

Do you just wish you could let it all go and feel clearer and more refreshed every day?

Then this book is for you!

I am going to share with you some of the MOST effective daily habits that you can add into your life to live longer, live happier and worry less!

I have given you the habit, along with an explanation and how you can apply them to *your* life immediately!

Also, ANYONE can benefit from these habits, whether you're experiencing just a little stress and worry, or completely drowned.

And, yes, they help reduce stress, but they also help you live a healthy life, as well as feel energized throughout your day!

What will this book teach you?

This book is not like others!

It doesn't just contain generic advice that we all already know, but actual stress-busting habits that have been identified to REDUCE stress levels, ELEVATE mood, IMPROVE energy levels, and LEAD to a more healthy life!

Some of these habits are very simple and you can begin implementing them today, and some are a little more difficult, in that you will need to practice them more!

I will also share with you why each of these habits work and are so effective – along with a simple action plan to help get you started and on your way to lasting success!

Introduction

Stress is a part of our everyday lives. It comes in many different forms whether it's a mean boss at work or daily arguments with your spouse. But what a lot of people don't seem to realize is how their simple everyday habits could be contributing to their high stress levels.

We all have negative habits that are not good for us. We tend to want to blow them off and not think about them because they make us more comfortable. These negative habits are actually addictions more than anything else. They are something we latch onto in order to get a little bit of relief from the pains and heartache of our stress.

The problem with addictions is they can be unhealthy. The most common negative addictions are overeating, junk food, smoking, alcohol, caffeine, and many others. We all know these things are not good for us, but yet so many people still use them for relief.

The relief you feel from these addictions will eventually turn into stress because you will be so dependent on them. Then like any drug, the more you take them the more you stress over wanting them.

Of course, negative habits don't just come in the form of drugs or stimulants. Sometimes it is simply how we are living our lives and acting towards others that contribute to our stress. The sad thing is many people don't even realize where there stress comes from.

We all come from different backgrounds and have a different perspective about the world and about life.

For some people, they have a positive spin on the world while others think negatively about it. These feelings and viewpoints will more than likely reflect on one's personality.

Those who think negatively all the time are constantly in a stress bubble. You will never see them happy because they are always angry with everyone.

If you were to ask them why they are so angry and stressed out, they probably couldn't give you an answer that breaks it all down. They would just say they are angry about everything in the world.

Healthy Habits

What you are going to learn from this book "Healthy Habits" is that you don't have to live your life feeling stressed out all the time. Not when there are ways to reverse the habits that are making you feel stressed out in the first place.

The key to reversing these bad habits is by replacing them with healthy habits, hence the name of the book.

Believe it or not, not all habits are bad for you. It is possible to develop positive habits that benefit your health.

How do you recognize positive habits versus negative habits?

For one thing, positive habits are not exactly addictive. Sure you may get used to performing these healthy habits after a while, but they are not something that you will stress out over if you cannot perform them.

On the other hand, negative habits will cause you to feel more stressful and will contribute to your poor mental state.

The book you are about to read goes over 17 healthy habits that will help you live longer, live happier and worry less. These three things are all interconnected.

If you reduce your stress levels then you will worry less. If you worry less then you will be happier, which will help you live a longer life because the stress won't be deteriorating your health anymore.

You may already have many of the healthy habits in this book, while others you may not have. As you go through the book, try and count how many of these healthy habits you have. If you find that you have the opposite habit, which is negative, then make note of that as well.

For example, the first chapter is about stopping your caffeine binge.

The negative habit here would be if you are currently drinking caffeine. The positive habit would be if you are currently not drinking caffeine.

The chapters are written under the assumption that you already have the negative habit. If you don't then just move on to the next chapter.

If you do then you will discover solutions on how to overcome the negative habit by turning it into a healthy one.

Try to go through each chapter one at a time. Even if you feel like you already have the healthy habit described in the chapter, read through it anyway because a refresher of why your healthy habit is important can never hurt.

Once you make it through the book, compare the number of healthy habits that you already have to the number of negative ones.

If the negative number is significantly higher then you know you have your work cut out for you.

But that is good because at least you now know where your stresses are coming from. This means you have already taken your first step towards recovery.

The next step is to take the advice in this book and try to fix the negative habits that you do have.

Do not expect it to be easy though because changing your habits never is. As human beings, we are often reluctant to accept change because it causes us temporary stress on top of the already existing stress.

What you have to realize is that changing yourself for the better will eventually take away both the temporary stress and the already existing stress. But first, you must know how to deal with the stress of change beforehand.

That is what this book will help guide you with.

Please note that all of the advice in this book is merely opinionated. This book was not written by a doctor or medical professional. So if you have uncontrollable stress or anger management, then it is always advised to seek care from a medical professional if you cannot handle it on your own.

Stress Buster 1

Stop the Caffeine Binge

Many of us lead very busy lives. In fact, it can get so busy and stressful that we hardly have time to sleep. This causes us to feel tired throughout the day, which ultimately affects our productivity at work or school.

People that wake up tired usually start their day by drinking a cup of coffee. They drink coffee because it almost immediately wakes them up after it is ingested. The secret ingredient in coffee that causes this effect is caffeine.

Caffeine is basically a drug that alters your central nervous system into an unnatural state. It temporarily boosts your level of focus and assertiveness, which allows you to feel less tired. This is supposed to help you get through your day without feeling groggy.

This "fake" level of energy is why caffeine consumption has gotten so out of hand. People simply like having a few cups of coffee in order to make up for the lousy sleep they had during the night. But this energy boost will not last forever and will eventually result in unwanted negative side effects.

When people feel these negative side effects, it will only cause them more stress because the positive effects will no longer exist anymore. Instead, they will be stuck with additional bad feelings that increase their stress and anxiety levels even more.

Adenosine Receptors

We all have something in our body called adenosine receptors. Our body produces adenosine as a way to tell the brain it is tired.

These receptors are all over our bodies, even in our muscles. So when we workout or simply work all day. These receptors get produced and tell the brain to rest.

People really misunderstand what caffeine actually does in your body. The reason why it is a "fake" energy boost is because it is not actually giving you energy. All it is doing is making you not feel tired anymore.

Caffeine is something that prevents the adenosine receptors from signaling to the brain that it is tired. Then as you continue to stay awake, more adenosine receptors build up in your body to try to get you to go to sleep. This is what eventually brings the caffeine "crash."

Once the effects of the caffeine wear off, it won't be blocking the adenosine receptors anymore. And because you built up so many receptors while you were on caffeine, now those receptors are going to go straight to your brain to signal that you need sleep. This will bring upon you an intense feeling to want to sleep, which is what the crash is all about.

So, imagine if you have a busy day and you start to crash around 12 noon. At this point, you will be stressing yourself out over trying to stay awake in order to complete the things you have to get done. Then either two things will happen. You will consume more caffeine to stay awake or you will sleep and not get any work done. Either way, it will increase your stress in the long run.

Some people are able to tolerate caffeine because they consume it in moderation. But for others, they develop a dependency on the drug and it causes them to overindulge in its consumption. If you find yourself depending on caffeine to stay awake, then you need to quit binging on it all together.

Caffeine Withdrawal

It is easy to tell an addict that they should just stop consuming caffeine if they want the negative symptoms to go away. While this would be the solution in a perfect world, we do not live in a perfect world.

People cannot just quit caffeine or any drug because someone tells them to. Instead, they need to strategize or even seek outside help to quit caffeine.

Most people can just strategize a way to quit caffeine. It is not such a harmful drug to the point where it will require you to go to rehab, like with cocaine or heroin. You just have to figure out how to rid yourself of all the foods and drinks that contain caffeine, or at least the ones with excessive amounts of it.

The number one drink that contains caffeine in it is coffee. Most adults will tell you they can't start their morning properly without that soothing cup of java to wake them up. Coffee has this effect because the average cup has 95 mg of caffeine in it.

This is three times the amount of caffeine that you would find in a cup of green tea or even a cup of soda.

What people don't realize from drinking coffee is that after a while, the effects of the caffeine won't be as beneficial anymore. In other words, they won't get as much energy from it as they used to get from just one cup.

This will make them want to have more cups of coffee in order to get that energetic buzz, which is what gives people the negative side effects of caffeine.

To overcome your caffeine addiction from coffee, you should replace your normal coffee with decaffeinated coffee. The idea here is that you will be tricking your mind into keeping up with the habit of having your coffee in the morning and throughout the day. The only difference here is the coffee won't have caffeine in it.

As you continue to drink decaffeinated coffee, you will notice that all of the negative symptoms from the caffeine will disappear. You will start feeling less irritable and have less anxiety as well. It will even get to a point where coffee will not be addictive anymore either because that caffeine drug was not being consumed.

Another way to overcome the addiction to coffee is to go with a drink that has less caffeine in it. For example, green tea contains about 30 mg of caffeine per cup. Not only that, it contains plenty of antioxidants that will clean out toxins and free radicals that cause cell damage within your body.

Since you will feel much better from drinking green tea, you won't even notice the negative side effects from consuming the small amount of caffeine. But at the same time, you will be feeding into that caffeine addiction in smaller amounts. This will help you gradually stop being dependent on it until you don't crave it ever again.

Discover Scientifically-Proven "Shortcuts" & "Hacks" to Lose Weight FASTER (With Very Little Effort)

For this month only, you can get Linda's best-selling & most popular book absolutely free – *Weight Loss Secrets You NEED to Know*.

Get Your FREE Copy Here:
TopFitnessAdvice.com/Bonus

Discover scientifically-proven tips to help you lose weight faster and easier than ever before. With this book, readers were able to improve their weight loss results and fitness levels. So, it's highly recommended that you get this book, especially while it's free!

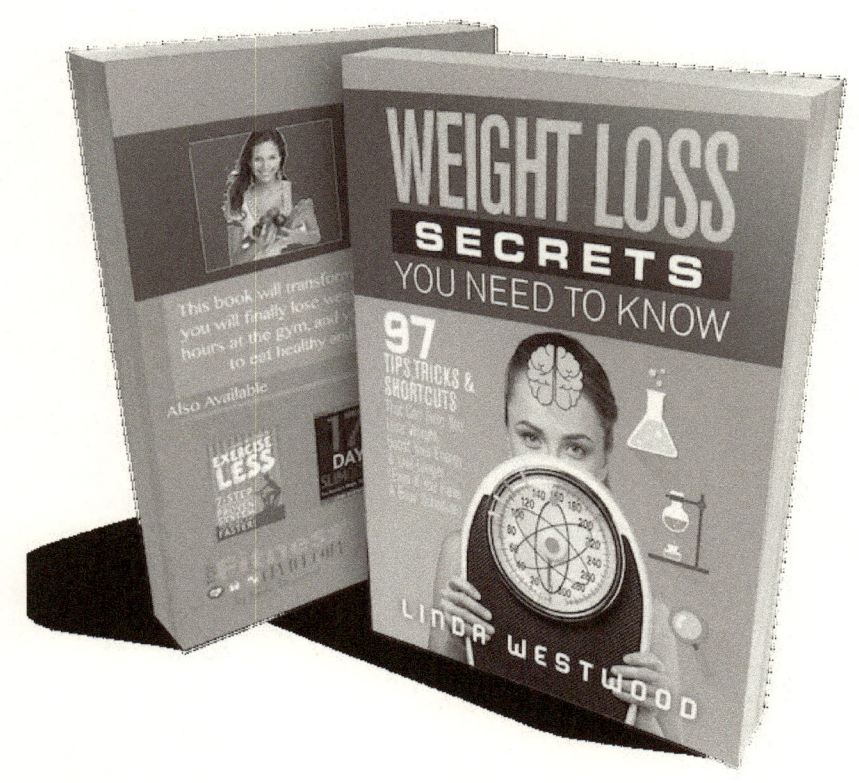

Get Your FREE Copy Here:

TopFitnessAdvice.com/Bonus

Stress Buster 2

Take Control of the Controllable

The things we experience in our lives often stay with us forever. It is easy for us to dwell on the past, especially on the negative things that might have happened. These are things that cannot be changed because nobody can change the past.

People often stress themselves out about things they have no control over, like mistakes they made in the past. They torture themselves with thoughts of wishing they had done something differently or wishing they could go back to change what they did wrong.

If you do not take control over your life in the present then nothing is ever going to get better. People sometimes have a tendency to think something is going to save them or someone will come along to help them gain control over their life.

The reality is that we are all in charge of our own lives. Sure there are people who may come along to lend us a hand, but in the end the weight of our burdens and our lives rests on our own shoulders.

If you fail to realize that then you will remain stressed out and miserable for the rest of your life.

What you have to realize is that the past is in the past. If you keep dwelling on it then you are only going to bring yourself further down into a state of anxiety and depression. These are two feelings that nobody wants to let into their life any more than they have to.

Make Peace with the Past

The present and the future are the only two things you have control over. If you've made past mistakes that you regret, then try working hard to not make any more mistakes in the present.

In order to effectively take control of your life, you must first make peace with the past. This doesn't mean you will forget about the past because that is impossible. Those memories will never go away. You only have two choices with the memories in your head. You can let them continue to bother you or you can accept them and move forward. Acceptance is simply telling yourself that what happened in the past… simply happened.

If you tell yourself that you learned from your mistakes and that you are a better person for what you did, then the past can always become a lesson learned. We all have to learn somehow and unfortunately, for most of us we learn from the mistakes we make.

Make a List of Controllable Situations

Acceptance of the past is the key to moving forward and gaining control over the present. Once you have gained acceptance, you need to carefully look at your life and the problems you are currently facing.

Make a list of everything in your life that currently makes you unhappy. This could be a bad job, unhappy marriage, weight issues and so on. All of these things are what you do have control over in the present. You just have to make the effort to change them for the better.

Make sure your list of things that you want to change is actually controllable. Don't put something ridiculous like "I want to be President of the United States" or "I want to win $1 million from the lottery."

These things are clearly uncontrollable. Sure if you want to be president you could go out and try to form your own campaign, but the decision for you to be president is still up to other people. Therefore, you don't have control over it.

Controllable situations are ones that affect you directly. There may be a few other people involved in the situation, but you must have some say in the outcome based on your actions. If you don't, then it is not controllable.

Of course, there are probably things in the present that cause you stress which you don't have control over. We all experience these things. But all you can do is to change what you have control over and learn to not stress out over the things you can't control.

Make the Change

Change can be a scary concept. It means taking yourself out of your comfort zone and trying something new. As humans, we often have trouble trying anything new. Our natural reaction is to feel scared and hold back. This is the feeling you have to push through.

Remember that people typically escape the present by drifting off into their imaginations or by thinking of the past. They wouldn't do this if their present was worth paying attention to.

You have to stop thinking about what you can't control anymore, such as events of the past or mistakes that you made which you regret. What's done is done. Now is time to move forward and change the controllable situations of the present.

How do you change the present? Well, take that list you made of everything that currently makes you unhappy in your life. Then start by trying to change one thing at a time on that list.

For example, let's say the first item you listed was ending a bad marriage. Instead of waiting for your spouse to die or leave you, try leaving them. Don't wait for somebody else to control your situation or pray to God for it to happen. You need to make it happen.

Every time you manage to change one thing in your life, cross it off your list and move down to the next thing you want to change on the list.

Keep going at this pace until you have successfully crossed off everything on the list and have totally changed your present. If you get to this point, you should be feeling very little stress because you will have the life you want to live.

There won't be any need to imagine a better life in the future or live in the memories of your past. Instead, the present will finally be worth focusing on. Then every time you a new situation arises that causes you stress, you can directly focus on changing that situation and every other one after that as they come.

Stress Buster 3

Emotional Eating the RIGHT Way

Obesity levels amongst people are certainly higher than they have ever been in history. This trend has spread throughout the world.

People are gaining weight at excessive rates. But the big question is, why? What is it that is really causing people to gain weight?

The quick answer is to blame it on the junk food, and that would be the logical answer. There are so many food manufacturing companies that are creating junk foods which are not healthy for people to consume.

Junk foods are basically processed foods that have been altered from their natural state. The common junk foods contain added pesticides, preservatives, flavorings, sugars, salts, seasonings and all kinds of things that are bad for our health.

Unnatural foods will cause you to feel unnatural. In other words, they will cause you to feel symptoms of stress, anxiety, irritation, irregular heart beat and more.

Even though these symptoms may be natural in some life circumstances, when they are caused simply by food then they are unnatural.

The Real Reason

We know junk food is the problem for the majority of health problems in America and other developed countries. Until government agencies ban junk foods from being sold in the supermarkets, they are always going to be there and people will always buy them.

It is no surprise to ordinary citizens that junk food is bad for them when they see it in the supermarkets. They know cookies, cakes, pizza, and fried foods are just going to make them feel lousy after they eat them. But they continue to eat these foods anyway. So again, why?

The real reason has to do with stress more than anything else. People live such stressful lives in the modern age. They have to worry about making a living, taking care of their kids and so on. It gets to a point where they really have no time to relax and feel comfortable at all.

People in stressful situations tend to form bad habits in order to relieve their stress. One of the biggest habits people develop is binge eating on junk food.

Once this happens, the unnatural chemicals and additives in those foods will raise their stress levels even higher. So instead of treating the problem, junk food just makes it worse.

Control the Eating

It is important that you understand the difference between emotional eating and regular eating. For example, if you are on a strict diet and you are able to control what you eat, this is regular eating.

When someone eats to relieve their stress and anxiety, this is emotional eating. Even someone who regularly sticks to a healthy diet regime could find themselves eating poorly if they are stressed. This is the inner demon that you have to learn to fight.

So, how does someone gain the discipline to control their eating under stressful situations? The first step is to try and distance yourself from all unhealthy foods. This means no filling your kitchen cupboards with junk food from the supermarket. Only fill your house with healthy foods. After all, if there are no healthy foods in your house then you won't be tempted to cheat.

Now if you are away from your house, like at work, then you might find vending machines nearby that will tempt you into eating poorly. These are always hard to resist for someone under distress.

Fortunately, there are certain types of foods you can eat beforehand that will help limit your cravings to relieve stress pains.

- **Avocados** – These are fruits that contain folic acid and vitamin B6. These nutrients have been scientifically proven to reduce stress levels by helping the central nervous system function well. It also contains potassium, which regulates blood pressure.

- **Salmon** – This type of fish is very high in omega-3 fatty acids, which can elevate you into a good mood. These acids also keep your heart strong, especially if your cortisol levels are high. These stress hormones get released under pressure and cause damage to your heart if they remain high. Omega-3s will prevent this.

- **Broccoli** – This vegetable is a good source of Vitamin C, which is what strengthens the immune system. When you feel stress and anxiety, it can put a burden on your immune system. It will even make you susceptible to colds and flu bugs.

- **Almonds** – These nuts are loaded with magnesium, which is a mineral that lowers cortisol levels. This will calm down the nervous system when it starts feeling stressed out. You will even sleep better as a result of eating these, which will then help you in other ways as well.

These are the four foods you should have on hand with you at all times, whether you are at work, school or wherever.

Two of these foods are so simple to carry that you don't even need to cook them.

As for the salmon and broccoli, just cook them beforehand and then bring them with you in a Tupperware container.

Now, every time you start feeling stressed out during the day, go ahead and eat a little bit of these foods. You don't necessarily have to eat bites from all of them, although that wouldn't hurt. If you are under time constraints and don't have time to eat, then almonds would be the best food to munch on.

Almonds are hard food and can conveniently be eaten from your desk at work or anywhere. Since they lower cortisol levels, this will ultimately be what you need to keep your stress under control. Then when you have your next lunch break, go ahead and eat the rest of the foods to further calm yourself down.

Now you can still eat other fruits and vegetables if these mood friendly foods don't fill you up. But just remember to stay away from all processed foods because they will reverse the positive feelings you have already endured from the healthier mood foods.

Eventually, you will start to develop a habit of controlling your mood through healthy eating every time you feel stressed out. Then it will become a routine for you, which means you will have successfully turned a bad habit into a good one.

I hope that you are enjoying this book so far, and if you could spare 30 seconds, I would greatly appreciate you leaving a review on Amazon.com.

Stress Buster 4

The ONE HABIT That WILL Extend Your Life

Physical activity is an important thing that should be incorporated into everyone's life. Unfortunately, people are not nearly as physically active as they used to be in our society. This is one of the main reasons why people's stress levels are so high these days.

Between the automobiles, planes, trains and other modes of transportation, people don't really need to walk around much anymore. They have vehicles that will take them anywhere they need to go.

Even most jobs today require people to sit in front of a computer or at a desk for an extended period of time. People don't really have opportunities to move their bodies anymore. And if they want to exercise, they are usually too busy to do that as well.

A lack of physical activity can cause many serious health effects later in life. After all, the human body is meant to move around. That is why we are born with two legs. If it doesn't move around then the body won't respond well.

Physical activity helps regulate blood pressure, heart rates, lung health, blood circulation, air circulation and more. Perhaps one of the most notable benefits of physical activity is weight loss. All of these things contribute to giving you a longer lasting life.

If you do not engage in consistent physical activity then you could eventually suffer a heart attack or stroke. Furthermore, you will feel sluggish and tired all the time as well. You might think physical activity is exhausting, but it can actually boost your energy levels if it is performed on a regular basis.

What is consistent physical activity?

When the phrase "physical activity" is used, it is easy to come up with your own idea of what it means. Physical activity for some means getting up and going to work each day. For others, it means exercising in a gym for at least 20 minutes per day.

Physical activity means to move your body around in order to perform an action. So when you are consistently active, this means you do not stop and take breaks in between the activity. In other words, you need to perform cardiovascular exercises for at least 20 minutes each day without a rest.

Cardiovascular activities are any exercise that consistently gets your heart rate up. The ideal amount of time to get your heart rate up is 20 minutes or more.

This amount will be just enough to keep your blood circulating and your heart healthy each day. You will also be able to breathe better in your lungs as well.

You don't necessarily have to get a gym membership to perform cardiovascular exercise. A simple 20-minute walk around your neighborhood each day will do just fine.

Combat Stress

You already know that exercise is the key to having a healthy body. But what you probably don't often think about is how exercise reduces stress levels in your body.

Do you ever notice how much better you feel after going on a long walk or run? Why do you think you feel that way?

The reason has to do with a chemical produced in your central nervous system called "endorphins."

Endorphins get released into the receptors of your brain to relax the body and eliminate feelings of stress. Exercise is the main way to get these endorphins released, so you can feel relaxed.

Therefore, the next time you feel stressed out about something, try consistent physical activity for 20 minutes. Then see if you still feel as stressed as you were before. Chances are you will feel much better.

If you are really stressed out and have more free time, think about increasing your amount of time spent on exercising. The more physical activity you perform, the more stress relief you will feel afterwards.

The Exercises

The best exercises that will keep you healthy are walking, jogging, running, cycling and swimming. If you are a beginner or haven't exercised in a long time, then start with a walking regimen. This will get your body used to moving around a lot without having too much intensity.

People who are obese often make the excuse that they can't go on walks because it is too painful for them to carry all their weight around. But like anything in life, if there's a will there's a way.

If you are severely obese or suffer from a disability that prevents you from moving your legs too much, then swimming is an available cardiovascular option. Swimming allows you to float and move around the water without needing your legs.

The real neat thing about swimming is it can make you feel lighter than you really are. When you swim most of your body will be floating on the water as you glide yourself forward with your arms. This will provide the exercise you need without straining your legs.

Now for all the rest who find walking regimens to be too easy, you can upgrade your exercise to jogging or running. Jogging is probably the best choice at first, so you can get used to moving at a faster pace.

As you get better at moving faster on your feet, you can start more running exercises to really boost up your metabolic rate and burn more fat off your body. It all depends on how far you want to take your exercise.

You don't necessarily have to keep improving your speed and the amount of time you spend exercising. If 20 minutes a day is all you can spare and you simply aren't into running or moving fast, then sticking with the walking is certainly better than nothing. It will still give you the health benefits you need.

It is recommended that you perform your physical activity in the morning or before you go to work. This will give you the required boost of energy you need to start your day. Think of it as a warm up for your job.

By using exercise as a natural energy booster, you won't feel compelled to drink caffeine or consume any other kind of unhealthy stimulant to wake you up.

Stress Buster 5

You Could Already Be Doing This WRONG

Sleep is something we all need in order to fully repair our bodies and energize it for the next day. If we do not get enough sleep then we won't have enough energy to complete the tasks we need to get done.

Health experts recommend that people get at least 8 hours of sleep each night in order to fully recharge itself.

However, most people lead such hectic lifestyles that they barely have time to sleep 4 hours a day. This will lead them feeling tired and unfocused when they wake up.

What is even worse is there are people who set aside 8 hours a day to get sleep, but still end up feeling tired in the morning. Why do you think that is? It mainly has to do with the quality of their sleep more than anything.

People rarely get a quality night's sleep these days. Usually there are distractions in the house that might wake them up, such as loud noises from dogs or children. This means they have to keep waking up and going back to bed, which ruins the quality of the sleep.

What you have to do is eliminate all bad habits that are causing you to sleep poorly. These habits involve food, sleeping position, and the pleasantness of your overall environment.

Eating Affects Sleep

Sleep is something that should be prepared for throughout the day. Everything from what you eat to the activities you've performed will contribute to the quality of your sleep.

So, if you've been eating pizzas, cakes and other junk foods, you will likely have an upset stomach which will keep you awake all night long.

It would be easier to get a good night sleep if you just stopped eating junk food all together. Not only would this help your quality of sleep, but it would provide other health benefits as well.

Let's just assume you have trouble in that department. You can still readjust your eating schedule so you don't feel as full at night. For example, it is better to eat your biggest meals after you just wake up. This way you will be active for a lot longer, which will help burn the calories.

At nighttime, this is when you should have lighter meals because you don't need as many calories for energy at this point in the day. So eat just enough food to where you won't be hungry anymore, but not full.

Now getting back to the diet, drinking water periodically throughout each day will greatly contribute to helping your digestive system process food better. This will reduce bloating and constipation while you are immobile during sleep.

There is a theory that eating right before sleep will cause you to stay awake. In actuality, it is just the opposite. It all depends on if you are hungry before you go to sleep or not.

If you had a light dinner then chances are you will feel a little hungry before bedtime. This is okay because you can just eat an extremely light snack, like Greek yogurt or a banana, to cure these hungry pains. You won't feel full from them either.

Along with your light bedtime snack, you should drink some herbal tea. Organic green tea is certainly the best because it will put you in a state of relaxation and help you fight toxins inside your body during the night.

Sleeping Position

Now if you are someone who sleeps poorly, but has 8 hours to spare and no distractions in the house, then your sleeping position is likely to blame.

People often sleep on their sides, which is actually very bad for the spinal and cervical posture of the body. This is also what causes back pains in individuals, especially older individuals.

These pains are what will keep somebody up all night long. There are two methods that could potentially help this situation.

The easiest method is to put a pillow between your knees while you sleep on your sides. This will help straighten out the alignment of your spine throughout the body.

The harder method is to sleep flat on your back, preferably without a pillow for your neck.

If you lie totally flat on the bed with no curves or pillows pushing your head up, this will even out your spine completely and prevent any more back pains from occurring.

Some people even try sleeping on the floor after they get used to sleeping flat on their bed. You can place a few comforters down on the floor to make the surface a little smoother on your skin. If you can maintain a straight posture on your back throughout the night, then you will feel great in the morning.

This method works well for some people, but others may find it too difficult. If that is the case then just stick with the pillow between your knees method. This will alleviate much of the tension on your back.

The Environment

We don't always have control over our environment. If we live in a rowdy neighborhood or big city, then you are likely going to hear noises from outside which will disturb your sleep. It is easy to say that you should just move, but that is not realistic for everyone.

The only environment you really have control over is the one inside your home. You need to do everything you can to keep the noise levels down, so you can sleep pleasantly.

If you live alone and have no kids, spouse or pets, then reducing the noise will be easy. But if you have anyone else in the house living with you then you will need to invest in some earplugs.

Earplugs are a great way to temporarily deafen yourself by sticking a plug into the ear canal of each ear. That way you won't hear anything throughout the night, even if there are noises present nearby.

Another way to create a pleasant environment is by turning on white noise. Studies have proven that white noise can block all other irregular sounds from around a room. Not only that, but white noise contains all the frequencies that can possible be heard at the same time.

White noise is able to stimulate the brain because it is one constant noise that has no variables. So the brain doesn't get distracted by any changes in sound waves or frequencies. This allows it to stay relaxed and not stress over any varying noises within the environment.

Stress Buster 6

Rest Your Mind Regularly

People are living busier lives now more than ever. Busy lifestyles tend to cause people to worry about a lot of different things. With so much on their minds, they tend to have more trouble focusing on the things currently in front of them.

When we worry about many things it causes stress and anxiety. People very rarely know how to deal with stress that involves the mind. Some might recommend taking a nap or doing something fun to forget about their problems. But the real solution has to do with resting the mind instead of the body.

Sure you can forget about your problems if you go to sleep and become unconscious. But those problems are going to still be there when you wake up. That is why you need to find a way to clear those problems from your mind. That way you can sleep better and focus better in your daily life.

In other words, you need to practice meditation on a regular basis.

Meditation

Meditation is one of the earliest forms of stress relief to ever exist. Once you have mastered it, you can control your thoughts by keeping out negative memories and focusing on positive ones.

For thousands of years, meditation has been practiced by people all around the world. It was used for getting in touch with the spiritual world and the mystical forces that inhabit it.

Back then, people thought the spirits were causing them to relax through the mediation. Now we know it is the mental tranquility aspect of meditation that helps relieve stress.

Meditation is the practice of training your mind to eliminate all thoughts, worries and desires. This puts you in a state of harmony where your mind is not exercising any brainpower or stressing itself out.

Along with reducing your negative emotions, you will also become more self-aware and more focused on the present things in your life. That way you don't keep dwelling on the past, and becoming stressed from your thoughts.

Meditation has also been known to help people with certain health disorders such as high blood pressure, depression, anxiety, heart disease and sleep problems. All of these disorders can be attributed to stress, which is what meditation relieves.

How to Meditate

Most people who have never meditated before only know what they have seen in the movies. After all, how many people in real life do you know who meditate? If you live in the western world, then you probably don't know anybody who mediates.

In the modern age, many people learn how to meditate simply by going online and learning about the various types of meditation. Each type has a unique way of putting a person in a state of mental tranquility. You are about to learn these meditation types now.

- **Guided Imagery** – It isn't always easy for someone to learn their minds and become mentally relaxed. They can't help but think of something. With guided meditation, you will focus on one image in your head and nothing else.

   The image in your head should be a positive one. It could be a place where you went on vacation or a situation that brings you pleasure. When you focus on this positive image, try to do more than just see it. Try to smell, hear and feel the environment of the picture as if you were really there.

   It helps to have another person guide you through the image by feeding you words about what you are seeing, hearing, and touching. If you don't have anyone like that, just keep practicing these techniques on your own.

- **Mantra Meditation** – When you practice mantra, you are repeating the same word over and over again to yourself. You don't say the word out loud. You just keep the word in your head and focus on repeating it in your mind.

   The idea here is that you won't be focusing on any other thoughts but the word. Make sure it is a calming word that brings you happiness or pleasure, like love or friendship.

- **Mindfulness** – This meditation is about being mindful, which means you are going to increase your awareness of the present and what is happening around you. This awareness could be everything from your surroundings to simply focusing on the flow of breath that comes out of your mouth. If any other thoughts outside of the present come into your head, you will just let them flow right back out of your head.

- **Yoga** – Here is something you have probably heard of before. Yoga is a unique form of meditation, but people often don't think of the mental side of it because yoga involves physical movements.

Yoga is a series of controlled postures and breathing exercises that allow your body to become more flexible. Once you have achieved flexibility, you will have a calm mind. The reason for this is because the yoga poses require strict concentration and balance in order to perform them.

What you are really learning from yoga is how to focus your body and mind to do whatever you want it to. Even though it helps you physically, you achieve a mental discipline from it too. You can use this discipline to help you focus more on good things and block out the bad things that cause you stress.

- **Zazen** – Zazen is derived from the ancient Buddhist traditions of meditation, which is now used in the more modern Zen traditions of Buddhism. It basically involves getting into a seated position and just sitting there for extended periods of time.

    This meditation also requires you to keep your back straight while you sit and just stare straight ahead. Zazen is the most difficult meditation to learn because you do not have to guide your breathing or pay any particular attention to just one thought.

Perform Meditation Regularly

Meditation is not a quick solution to curing your stress. Sure it can eliminate it in the moment, but if you don't regularly meditate then your stress will come back.

Negativity is all around us and it is easy to focus on it if you don't meditate often. It is similar to how somebody who doesn't exercise often will get fat as a result. You have to keep up the exercise in order to keep the fat off.

Meditation has to be done at least three times per week to effectively train your mind to keep out negative thoughts. It doesn't really matter which meditation type you perform. Just pick one that you are most comfortable with and go for it.

If you want to challenge yourself, try out a new form of meditation after you have mastered another one. You may discover a new type of meditation that works better for you.

Meditation should be performed for at least 30 minutes. However, if you are in a state of mental tranquility then you are probably not going to be concerned about the time. You could always set an alarm on your phone if you really have to watch your time. Otherwise, just enjoy the peace of mind and mental escape that meditation offers.

Once again, thank you for reading this book, and I hope you're getting a lot of valuable information. I would greatly appreciate it if you could take 30 seconds to leave me a review for this book on Amazon.com.

Stress Buster 7

Rest Your Body Regularly

You have already learned that sleep is essential for maintaining a healthy body. Sleep provides the body with a chance to repair its cells and tissues. It also reenergizes the body so it will have enough energy to get through the next day.

Have you tried all of the methods of sleeping better that were previously mentioned in this book? Are you still having trouble sleeping?

There may be one essential element to sleeping better that you still haven't tried.

People who are physically and emotionally stressed out will need a massage in order to sleep better. You are probably familiar with what massages are. It is when someone gently uses their hands and fingers to loosen up the aching muscles in your body.

People who are stressed out often have tense muscles that need to be loosened. This will help reduce their stress levels, improve circulation in the muscles, lower blood pressure and release all the inner tension that has been bottled up inside.

Those who suffer from arthritis, headaches, lower back pain or sports injury will also benefit from a massage. It will ease the painful symptoms to the point where they can sleep at night without the pain of their condition waking them up.

Have you ever gotten a massage? It is surprising, but when you ask most people if they have ever gotten a massage they will say no. Of course, this doesn't refer to having your spouse or partner rub your shoulders. You need a professional who understands the chemistry behind massages.

Besides easing the tension in your muscles to help you sleep, massages help the body release a chemical called serotonin. This is a chemical in the brain that regulates the sleep cycle of the body.

People who lack in serotonin will experience insomnia or trouble sleeping. Massages will be the cure for this.

Massage Therapists

A true massage is performed by a massage therapist or someone who knows how to soothe tense muscles. For this, you usually have to go to school or get trained by another professional in massage therapy.

But you are not interested in becoming a massage therapist. You are interested in having one relieve your stress and the tension in your muscles. Therefore, you need to find a massage therapist to help you out by giving you a massage.

Both men and women are massage therapists. A male therapist is called a masseur and a female therapist is called a masseuse. Some people prefer certain genders massaging them for a variety of reasons.

Masseurs typically have stronger hands, so they can really soothe out the muscles and relax them better. On the other hand, some clients don't feel comfortable having a man touching them on their body. So, they have a masseuse do the massage instead.

Both kinds of massage therapists will do a great job, so it is really a personal preference more than anything.

Massage therapists are all over the place. You can just pick up the classified ads section of your local newspaper and check under the "Business Services" heading. Massage services are usually listed here.

The price of a massage session depends on who you hire. Message therapy is typically a private practice, so the therapists get to choose their own prices.

The average price for a one hour session is $75. You may think that is a lot of money, but a one hour massage will definitely release the built-up tension inside your body.

You only need to get a massage at least once every month. For those with lots of built up tension, you might want to get massages once a week to start. Then as you become more relaxed, you can move on to once a month.

Massage Types

There are basically four types of massages that will help you get a good night sleep by reducing your stress. Usually it is up to the massage therapist to choose the right one for you, depending on your condition.

- **Deep Massage** – This technique uses forceful hand strokes that move in a slow pattern. They target the muscle and connective tissues deep within your body. For anyone with muscle damages for working out in the gym or an injury, deep massages work best.

- **Swedish Massage** – This massage is very gentle on the muscles. It uses long relaxing strokes, vibration, kneading, deep circular movements and light tapping. People tend to feel energized after a good Swedish massage.

- **Trigger Point Massage** – People with tight muscle fibers will need this massage. It targets these tight fibrous areas of the muscles and helps ease the tension.

- **Sports Massage** – This is sort of a modification of the Swedish massage. It uses the same techniques, but is designed to specifically help heal people who have sports injuries or to help prevent them from occurring.

- **Aromatherapy Massage** – This massage uses scented plant oils on the skin which contain natural healing agents. These oils will energize the body and reduce stress levels. The most common oil used in this type of massage is lavender.

- **Shiatsu** – This is a Japanese style massage that uses finger pressure as a form of acupuncture on the body.

The finger pressure is applied in various sequences and held at each point for up to 8 seconds.

Shiatsu improves a person's energy flow and to regain mental balance in their life. When you first get Shiatsu done, you might feel like it is a little rough with the pressure. But when it is all done, you won't feel any soreness or tension at all.

- **Foot Massage** – Foot massages are not just something you see in the movies. They can actually be very beneficial to your body because there are certain foot points that correlate to various systems and organs within the body.

Extra Tips

You will see a lot of massage products advertised in the stores and on television. They are basically little vibrating machines that you put up against your back to relieve tension.

While you might feel a little something from a vibrating machine, it is not nearly as powerful and thorough enough to target tense muscle fibers and get them loose.

What you can do is study the previous chapter that talks about how to sleep better. It truly coincides with the information in this chapter about massages.

If your sleep position is good and you are in a relaxed environment, then these things will already help you ease tension on their own. Massages will only add additional support to all of that, but it won't do it alone.

If you are still experiencing a noisy environment or sleeping on your side, then take care of these issues first before turning to massages as a way to treat your sleeping troubles.

Stress Buster 8

Read Every Day

Millions of people, especially Americans, watch television every single day. In fact, studies show that the average American watches around 8 hours of television each day. That comes out to 56 hours of television per week, which are more hours than most people work each week.

Think about all the wasted hours we have spent in our lives watching television. Chances are they were not educational shows. Instead we are hooked on reality television, game shows, and sitcoms that really do nothing but make us sit back and forget about our own lives.

The only reason people watch so much television in the first place is because they are unhappy with their lives and they want to forget about it by living vicariously through others. It is through the lives of people on television that they get their satisfaction in life.

The problem with gaining happiness from television is that the happiness is only temporary. If you zone out and pretend to be someone you are not, eventually you are going to have to come back to reality and face your life. This is when you will become stressed.

The more television you watch, the more stressed out you get because you end up not doing anything to change your life for the better. Then when you look around you realize that you are much older and have still not done anything yet. This will be what ultimately pushes you over the edge.

Replace Television with Books

Think about how many hours per week that you spend watching television. What would you do with those hours if you weren't watching them? In the old days before television ever existed, people read books to keep themselves entertained.

Books can offer a lot of great benefits that television will never even come close to offering. For one thing, books allow you to enhance your imagination a lot more than motion picture can. When you read the words from a book you have to create the images of the words in your head. This makes someone more imaginative.

The best part about using your imagination from reading is that you have control over the images that you see in your mind. This creates a mental exercise that keeps the brain thinking and working itself. This will ultimately help you think better in general.

When we watch television, we are basically sitting in front of it without really thinking at all. Since the visual images are given to us, we don't have to use our minds to create them.

In fact, we don't really use our minds at all while watching television. This is ultimately the reason why constant television watching will reduce your intelligence.

So by incorporating books into your free time, you will become smarter and you will learn more in the process.

Beating the Habit

It can be challenging to turn away from television if you are already hooked on it. Most of us have been raised on television and we are used to it.

On the other hand, books have always been viewed as a nuisance because our teachers in grade school used to force us to read. So psychologically, we tend to keep viewing books as something boring because that was how we felt as kids.

No one ever teaches children about how to make reading fun. After all, you cannot expect a child with a short attention span to read a book if there is a television nearby.

Everywhere you go you will see televisions playing somewhere. They exist in bars, restaurants, hospital waiting rooms and every house in America. They even exist in schools where kids are told to read! So, how do you get away from them all?

The first thing you have to do is get rid of any televisions that exist in your house. This is obviously where the biggest temptation to watch it is going to be.

If you already have your television then you can sell it on eBay or through Craigslist. If you have to, give it away to your neighbor. Just make sure all televisions are out of your house. This may feel weird in the beginning because a house without television is so unheard of in our modern age. But this will be the key to overcoming your bad habit.

Once the television is gone, try going to a book store and filling up your shelves with books. You can choose any kind of books that interest you. These could be historical books, horror novels or anything.

Of course, it would be best to read something that will teach you new things because knowledge can only help you in life. However, you may find educational books to be boring in the beginning. In this case, pick a fictional novel that will excite you.

Now when you go out to public places you might want to carry a book around with you. That way if there is a television nearby, you can take out your book and start reading.

You could also use an Amazon Kindle device, which is an electronic eBook reader that can hold hundreds of books inside one tiny mobile device. This is definitely something you will want to invest in.

Remember the whole idea here is to exercise your mind and to use your imagination. These things will ultimately help you expand your mind and accomplish your goals.

Furthermore, it will reduce your stress levels in the process because you won't be thinking about your own personal problems. Instead you can distract yourself with reading material that will enhance your cognitive function.

And when it comes to your children, try to keep them away from television for their own sake as well. That way when they get older, they won't have to struggle with quitting television just like you have to.

More importantly, it will allow your children to fill their minds with whatever their imagination contains. They won't be subjected to television shows that contain violence and horrific images.

Believe it or not, these images create tension in people and actually contribute to their stress. Remember this every time you go to pick up the remote and you will successfully beat the bad habit of watching television.

Enjoying this book?

Check out my other best sellers!

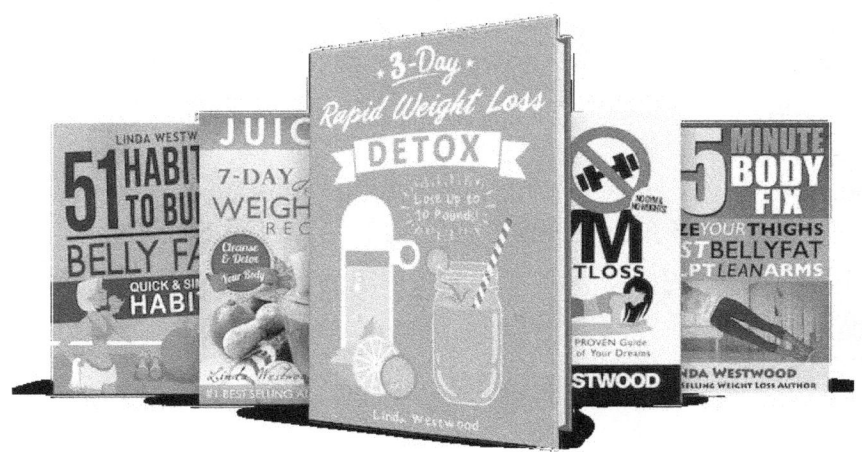

Get your next book on sale here:

TopFitnessAdvice.com/go/books

Stress Buster 9

Shift Negative Hobbies

The technological age has its ups and downs. The ups are the speed and convenience of communication that technology has given us. People are now able to talk, write and research faster than they ever could throughout history.

Unfortunately, technology has also caused a lot of people to develop negative hobbies as well. These are hobbies that are unproductive and simply take time away from doing things that could better your life.

The common negative hobbies that people have today are watching television, surfing the internet, playing video games, and texting on their Smartphone. It is easy for hours to go by without even realizing it while performing these activities.

All of these wasted hours could have been spent doing something more productive, like education, exercise or work. Then when you look back and realize how much time you wasted, you won't have much time left to perform the important tasks in your life.

Stress will eventually derive from negative hobbies because you will realize how much time you really did waste, which will cause you to get depressed. These negative hobbies have even come between family members. Don't let the same thing happen to you.

Substitution

This whole book is about substituting negative habits for positive ones. If you have made it this far in the book then you should already have some discipline for making changes in your life. This is good because you will need to make more changes with your negative habits

In the last chapter, you already learned that it is better to replace your time watching television with time reading books. You can do this simply by getting rid of your television. However, there are still other bad habits that drain hours from your life that you have to work on.

Let's start with sitting at a desk and going on the computer. Now this is a tough one because computers do have their essentialness in life. Computers allow us to budget our money, communicate with friends, and even read books. So you won't be able to just get rid of it that easily.

But even if you are being productive on the computer, you still need to spend some time away from it. Our physical bodies are not meant to sit in one place for too long. We need to get up and move around in order to stay healthy.

So here's what you can do. Every time you get the urge to do something unproductive on the computer, like playing video games or watching porn, turn off the computer immediately and go for a walk outside.

The outside world is a big place and there are literally dozens of activities you can perform that are more exciting than sitting in front of a computer playing World of Warcraft.

You can go for a walk, swim at the beach, take a bike ride on a trail, and more. Just perform some type of physical activity each time you get the urge to be unproductive.

Eventually, you will train yourself to stop being unproductive by switching gears and doing something else that will benefit you. Exercise is definitely the best thing for your physical wellbeing.

Socialize and Dating

If you are single then you probably watch television and go on the internet just to fill your free time. This could potentially cause you to become antisocial and develop even more bad habits.

To better fill your free time, try going out on more dates. If you are a shy person who doesn't know how to ask someone out, then try using online dating websites to arrange a meet up.

This might sound hypocritical because you were just told not to go on the internet. However, if you use the internet to find a real-life date then you will still be productive. Then once you find someone to date, you can focus on them and not on the internet.

The point here is to try to replace your negative habits of isolation with positive habits of socializing. Sure you can exercise to replace these negative habits, but there is only so much exercise you can perform in one day. Eventually, you will have to find another good habit to replace the bad ones with.

The relationships you form don't necessarily have to be romantic ones either. The ability just to form new friendships is better than sitting at home in isolation. Then the more friends you make, the more opportunities you will have in the future to get out of the house and away from those addictive electronics.

Last Resort

You might be saying to yourself, "I like to play video games, watch movies and surf the internet. I am not going to change." Well if this is your attitude, then turning those bad habits into something good.

When it comes to video games, there a number of interactive games out that require people to physically movie their bodies in order to control the action. A popular game is Wii Boxing for the Nintendo Wii.

This is a game that keeps you standing on your feet and makes you simulate punches to control the boxing of the game. After about 30 minutes of playing this game, you will surely be out of breath.

The point here is you should incorporate video games that do something good for you, like exercise. If you have educational video games that stimulate your mind, then you should try those out as well.

As for television, why spend so much time sitting on the couch while you watch it?

Instead you should purchase a treadmill and put it in your living room. Then every time you watch television, start walking on the treadmill for at least 3 mph.

Like with the video games, you are incorporating exercise into your television watching habits. That way you can physically benefit from watching it. You may also find gyms with small televisions attached to treadmills. The same concept can apply here as well.

Now surfing the internet may be hard to incorporate exercise with, unless you are watching a fitness video and are going to perform along with it. There are plenty of free fitness videos on YouTube and Bodybuilding.com.

So if you feel like you want to kill a few hours on the internet, try turning it into something beneficial by educating yourself on something new or physically learning a new exercise.

Others who are considering purchasing this book would love to know what you think. If you could spare a few seconds, they would greatly appreciate reading an honest review from you. Simply visit the page on Amazon.com.

Stress Buster 10

Be Realistic About Time

Time is something that many of us take for granted. We fill our time with all kinds of things, like work, school, entertainment, socializing and sleep.

But, how much time do we actually waste on things that are unproductive? You need to be realistic about your time if you are ever going to accomplish anything.

When we are young it seems like time lasts forever. But as we get older time, time flies by so quickly that we don't even realize it. For those who don't have time management skills, they could easily set unrealistic goals for themselves every day.

When you set unrealistic goals for yourself it could end up causing you stress while trying to achieve them all. Then when you don't achieve them, you will feel even more stress and anxiety.

Instead of backing off and cutting your schedule to reduce the stress, you will be tempted to overload your schedule even more to make up for the time that you already wasted. You have to prevent yourself from getting into a cycle like this.

Shorten To-Do List

You need to get realistic about your time and the amount of work you can handle with it. We all want to achieve lots of things quickly, but there is only so much you can do in one day.

If you have a to-do list then take a look at how many tasks you have set for yourself each day. Now mark down how many of these tasks you have actually accomplished. Were you able to complete them all?

If the answer is no, then you obviously set too many tasks for yourself each day. Therefore, you need to limit the tasks on your list so you can complete them all within those days.

Now you might be saying to yourself, "I have too much responsibility and I cannot afford to shorten my to-do list." Really, so is everything on your list essential in your life?

If your list pertains to your job, then you will definitely need to learn to delegate responsibilities to other people. Do you think managers do everything by themselves? That is why they hire employees in the first place.

As for lists that pertain to personal tasks, these are usually easier to adjust if you simply try. The personal tasks of most people involve taking care of their kids, mowing the lawn, getting an oil change, and so on.

When you go down your to-do list spread out the tasks that don't have to be accomplished on any particular day. Obviously, picking up your kids from school or cooking dinner for your family is a necessity.

But when it comes to household chores or going out to eat, these are things that are not crucial and can be done when you have free time available.

If anything, have your kids help you with the chores if they need to get done and you don't have time to do them. In a way, family can be just like employees in a sense. Delegate the responsibility wherever you can and let your family help you out. That way you can relax more.

Make Your List a Priority

You have already learned about how wasting time can take away from performing your responsibilities. If you have a big to-do list and yet you find yourself watching television, then obviously you are not taking your time seriously.

Time goes by in a heartbeat. If you sit down and watch television, you could be wasting many hours without even realizing it. You may tell yourself that you'll still have time to get your workload done, but why put yourself under that strain?

If you leisurely ignore your workload with the attitude that you'll get it done, then you are only going to add more stress to yourself trying to get it done in a shorter amount of time. So, why waste time?

What you need to do is perform all of your duties and alleviate your workload first. If you are able to do this then you can spend the rest of your time relaxing in front of the television and rewarding yourself that way. But, you must always make your to-do list a priority.

Limit your Responsibilities

There are some people who simply cannot handle too much stress. One example is someone who has an important job while trying to raise a family at the same time. These are too many responsibilities for one person to handle.

For some people, they may not be able to shorten their to-do list because they have so many important responsibilities. If this is the case in your situation and you cannot handle them, then you might want to think about getting a less responsible job.

People are so hungry for success these days that they forget about living a quality life. This doesn't necessarily mean working 80 hours a week and trying to get rich. It just means being comfortable and happy with your position in life.

So if you work a demanding job, then try to take another position that is less demanding. Then you won't have to stress out over time anymore.

Say "No" to New Tasks

The final thing you need to remember is not to pile on more work on top of the work you already have. If you know you are swamped with a heavy workload, then you need to refuse anymore work.

There is no sense in trying to satisfy everyone all the time when it creates an unsatisfactory life for you. After all, these other people don't care about your stress levels. So you need to manage them on your own by easing the workload.

With personal tasks, it is easy to refuse those. As a parent, you can just tell your kid "no" and they have to accept it. This may not be as easy to do with your boss though. However, you have to be honest with them as well.

If you agree to anything your boss says, even though you don't have time, then you are going to end up doing a lousy job. Then that will make you look even worse in their eyes. It is better to honestly tell them you are too busy.

Stress Buster 11

Let Others Help You!

Independence is a trait that many of us possess in the modern age. We all want to feel like we can do everything ourselves because depending on others can become a hassle if you have issues with trust.

When you are at work, especially if you are a manager, then you likely cannot do everything by yourself.

This is why managers hire employees because they help do the work for them and increase productivity for the company.

But there are people who simply want to do everything on their own. This is a bad habit to get into because it creates additional pressure and anxiety from worrying about everything that you have to get done.

If you try to do everything by yourself then you are going to stress yourself out with all the heavy workloads. There is only so much burden that one can handle before they snap. Don't let this happen to you.

That is why teamwork and depending on others can help alleviate these stressful symptoms.

No one should have to feel like they need to do everything by themselves. All it takes is trust and delegation.

Get Help at Work

No matter what your problems are in life, you should always have at least one person around to help you figure them out. It is human nature to interact with others and work together.

When you are at a job then it is easy to ask for help because there are other workers around you who are familiar with your situation. Whether you are a manager or minimum wage laborer, you should always ask for help if you need it.

You might feel like asking for help is a sign of weakness, but it is not. The true weakness is holding back and not asking for help when you really need it.

The result of not asking for help will just create more problems in the workplace because you will have trouble completing your workloads and it will eventually be noticeable to others.

So you have to hold in your pride and seek help from whoever is available. Then you can the peace of mind of knowing that you did everything you could to do the job right. Best of all, this will relieve your stress levels.

To recap, managers can delegate their responsibilities to their other workers and get help that way. Then if the workers need help, they can ask their managers for assistance and they will provide it to them.

So no matter what, seeking help will always be the best way to approach any stressful work situation.

Personal Problems

But in our personal lives, that is a different story. Personal problems are the number one area where people don't want to ask for help. Some famous examples of this are dysfunctional marriages, abuse, homelessness, and so on.

People generally have too much pride to ask for help with their personal problems. But sometimes, we all need a helping hand when it comes to fixing a bad situation in our lives.

If you have family and friends then you are already in a great position to get help. Family and friends are a necessity in life that we often take for granted. They will be there for you and help you out with your problems the best they can.

You may feel like your family and friends won't be understanding about your problems. This is a common reason why people don't confide in their loved ones, but they must.

If they truly care about you then they will help you. So, don't be afraid to ask them for help. But if your problem is directly related to your family, then ask a friend for help. If your problem is with a friend, then ask a family member. Either way, there is always an option.

Now in extreme circumstances where you don't have any family or friends to turn to, your only alternative is to seek help from an outsider. This is somebody who you don't even know, but are forced to put your faith into.

If you have an emergency, the outsiders could be police, social services or any civil servant whose job is to help people in dire situations. They are all just one phone call.

For non-emergencies, you are probably looking for advice or guidance in how to accomplish something. There is nothing wrong with going on the internet and visiting a forum or message board for advice. Most people will be kind enough to give you free advice and help you with your problem.

Just remember to try to get help from someone. Otherwise, you will be dealing with the issues on your own and this will only cause you more stress. Asking for help in any situation reduces stress to at least some degree.

Eliminate Fear to Ask

As you can see, there are ways to get help in all situations. But it is up to you to actually put your pride aside and ask for help. Don't expect someone to come along and help you on their own because it almost never happens that way.

If too much pride is not your problem, then it most likely has to do with shyness. Sometimes people are just too introverted to really seek out help from people.

People become introverted for a number of reasons. Maybe they are depressed or just don't like being around people. Whatever the reason is, this can be a handicap to those who want to ask for help but are too afraid to.

So how do you eliminate this fear and ask for help when you need it? This is a psychological hurdle more than anything. The easy answer to this problem would be to seek therapy.

Most of the time, social anxiety issues occur in people with low self-esteem. In this case you should refer back to the chapters that talk about exercise and eating right. Not only will these things reduce stress, but they will make you feel better about yourself as well.

Then, perhaps, you will increase your self-confidence and have the courage to ask for help when you need it. All of these things are interconnected, so it could work for you.

Stress Buster 12

Hang Out with Family & Friends

There are two big reasons as to why people get stressed or have difficulties in their life. Chances are they either hang out with the wrong people or they just keep everything bottled up inside without talking to someone they can trust.

For those who have nobody to talk to, stress comes from mere loneliness and isolation. Human beings were not meant to be isolated creatures. It is an unfortunate thing in our society today where so many people shut themselves off from others out of fear or distrust.

As for those who do have families and friends, they may not necessarily be the best role models in our lives. It would be easy to say that if you have a problem then you should just talk to your friends or family members about it. But in some cases, they might not be the best people to talk to.

We all come from different families and different backgrounds. Some of us have family members who we can confide in and some of us do not.

For some, they have family members who are a negative influence and create more stress than there should be.

Those who have endured negativity from others in their lives are the ones who tend to isolate themselves because they are afraid of getting hurt again. But in reality, they are only hurting themselves by staying away from people and being lonely.

The trick is to find the right people and be happy with them.

Family and Friends

There are all kinds of people in this world. Some are positive and some are negative. If you happened to be in a situation where negative people surround you, then you shouldn't jump to conclusions and assume all people are like that. You just have to go out and find positive people.

Now if you do have family and friends who are loving and supportive, then great. You should hang out with them every chance you get when you are feeling bad about life or simply stressed out.

Friends and family who are positive will inflict their positivity onto you. Then you will feel better about your life and realize that your problems aren't worth stressing out over.

Hanging out with family and friends could mean having dinner with them or simply getting together for a chat. What you shouldn't do is get together and watch a movie on television. This is not communication.

The idea here is to engage in a conversation with your family and friends when you are feeling stressed. Sometimes a good talk goes a long way in reducing stress levels.

Meet New People

People who are negative often make excuses about why they are stressed out. The main excuse is that other people are nasty to them, so they will be nasty back. This will just turn you into a nasty person. Then when somebody positive comes along in your life, they won't want to be around you because your negativity is hurting their mood.

You need to break this cycle by getting away from the people who are a negative influence. Whether it is the people in your neighborhood or even the people in your family, you need to move to a new area immediately.

Moving to a new area gives you an opportunity to make new friends. Since nobody knows who you are there, you can totally reinvent yourself by not being a negative person anymore. No one will notice the difference if they don't know you. So don't be afraid to try.

With a fresh start, you can be positive to everyone you meet. Chances are this positivity will be reinforced back to you as you begin to meet new people. Then you will have a whole group of friends who you can now socialize with.

There are many ways to meet people. Besides at work, you can go to the gym or simply introduce yourself to somebody out in public. If you have neighbors then try to make friends with them as well. The more friends you make, the better you will feel about yourself.

Just make sure the people you make friends with are a positive influence. If they are not, then don't give them another minute of your time.

Social Schedule

You don't have to only hang out with people when you are feeling lousy. That will make your friends think you are a drama queen all the time. Not only that, but they will feel like you are only using them for comfort.

It is always a good idea to socialize with the positive people in your life on a regular basis, whether you are happy or sad.

Socializing is something we need in our lives as much as food because it keeps us alive and brings happiness.

Make a schedule or plan to go out with your friends at least a few days during the week. Once you do, you will notice that your mood will be elevated towards a more positive light. Then after a while, you will just become a more naturally happy person

Think about all the happy people you have ever met in your life, how many of them were loners? The answer is probably zero.

Loners are never really happy because they have no social schedule. Happy people tend to go out and mingle all the time. Now you know why.

No More Worries

One of the biggest benefits to socializing is that it takes your mind off your worries. Sure, you could watch television to get the same benefit, but you still won't feel too good.

In fact, you will feel a whole lot worse because you are not getting any positive reinforcement from other people. This is what you need to become happy yourself, which is something television cannot provide.

With the distraction that socializing provides, you will not worry so much anymore. Then you will feel less stress and have an increase in mental clarity. This is a good feeling.

I hope you have learned something from this book so far and would greatly appreciate it if you could leave an honest review on Amazon.com.

Stress Buster 13

Get Things Done NOW

How often have you put things off in your life? This could be putting off going to school, getting a job, or simply performing some task that you need to get done.

We are so used to telling ourselves, "I'll get to it later" because we don't feel like doing it right now in the present. This could be out of laziness or due to time constraints. The longer we put something off, the more stress it will cause us because we will keep thinking about having to get it done. Not only that, but we will obligate ourselves to perform more tasks that we will put off as well.

It will get to a point where you have a big list of things that you have to get done and because the list keeps getting bigger, you keep putting more things off. You need to stop this trend before it drives you insane.

Procrastination is the word that describes people who put things off until the last minute. Many of us were guilty of this in our grade school days. When the teacher would give an assignment, we would wait until the night before it was due to actually complete it.

Unfortunately, people carry over their procrastinating attribute into adulthood, which is where it causes them a whole lot more trouble. Adults have more responsibilities and so putting them off until the last-minute causes more stress.

If you were to procrastinate at work, for example, then it could ultimately lead to your termination if you are unable to get it done on time. But even if you get it done, you still have to stress yourself out over getting it done on time.

Don't Procrastinate

It would be simple to tell you "don't procrastinate" in order to achieve your goals and reduce your worries over getting things done. But, you have to really work at it because procrastination is usually a character flaw.

The first thing you should work on is not putting things off that you can easily accomplish in the present. For example, if you have a ¼ tank of gas and you drive by a gas station, don't talk yourself out of getting gas because you don't feel like stopping. Instead go forward and put more gas in your car.

Another example is fixing things around the house. If you have a wife and she tells you to replace the batteries in the smoke alarm, don't tell her you'll do it tomorrow or some other day. Do it immediately!

You need to get into the habit of doing mediocre tasks right away. These are things you really have no valid excuse to avoid, so don't make any excuses. Just get in the habit of doing things in the present.

If you need help getting into the habit, try to develop a reward system for yourself. You may even want to have your spouse help you with this if you have one.

Make an arrangement with your spouse so that every time you do something right away, then you will be treated with a reward. This could be a free dinner or a night out on the town.

Even if you don't have a spouse and you are trying to accomplish your own personal goals, you can still reward yourself in a similar fashion.

Let's say your car desperately needs an oil change because you've gone way over 3000 miles since your last one. What you could do is plan a day where you take your car in for the oil change and then buy yourself a Chinese food lunch afterwards. This will get you excited about accomplishing your task.

Rewards can come in all shapes and sizes though. They don't always have to be something where you spend money. You could reward yourself with sleep, television or anything that allows you to relax and feel good.

What will really make you feel good is to know that you have accomplished your goals. So even if you break a good habit by watching television, you would have still gotten your immediate tasks completed. Then you won't be stressed out as a result.

Schedule Big Events

Now there are certain events or goals in life that can't just be done right away. For example, if you have always wanted to take a vacation to Italy, you obviously can't just drop everything and go there immediately. You need to arrange it with your boss at work and with your family.

Therefore, what you should be doing is scheduling these goals in the present. Figure out right now when the best time would be to plan your event, whether it is a dream vacation or starting your own business.

Once you figure out a date in the near future that when you want to start your event, the next thing you have to do is take steps in preparing for the event.

If you are preparing for a trip then this would involve getting a passport, calculating costs, saving money, purchasing airfare, making hotel reservations and so on.

If you are starting your own business then you would start by writing a business plan, obtain a loan and choose a location for the establishment.

The point here is that you need to set a goal for yourself in the future and then spend all of your free time in the present working towards that goal.

You will be amazed how much more work you can accomplish towards your goal by having it scheduled out. Then you will feel good about yourself while knowing you are making an actual attempt to make your big goal a reality.

Stress Buster 14

Alter Your Mind

Are you the type of person that always focuses on the negative? If you are, this means you constantly think of the worst thing that can happen in every situation.

People who think the worst are usually trying to predict all the bad things that can happen, so they won't be surprised or shocked when they do happen.

The problem with thinking negatively all the time is that it makes you have a negative attitude, which will cause you to be apprehensive towards every situation. This ultimately leads to anxiety and worrying.

Not only that, but you will constantly be in a bad mood as well. Then people won't want to be around you, which will create even more tension.

It is very stressful to look for the bad in every situation. In order to overcome this, you must first realize that life is unpredictable. Otherwise, you are going to drive yourself crazy by worrying about everything that could happen badly in your life.

Focus on Positive Things

What you need to do is focus on the positive things in your life. Then when you are in a situation that is negative, just remind yourself of the good things you still have and let that get you through your bad times.

It would even be a good idea to make a list of all the good things in your life. That way if you have trouble thinking about them on the spot, you can refer back to the list and remind yourself of how lucky you really are.

Also, when you make a mistake in life you should think of it as a lesson learned. There are so many mistakes that you can make, such as getting into a bad relationship, running a red light and so on.

If you keep dwelling on those little mistakes you made then it will drive you crazy. Instead of dwelling on those mistakes, think of them as a learning experience for the future. Now those mistakes turned into a positive experience in that aspect.

You see there is something good in everything. You just have to focus on the good and stop swelling on the bad. That is how you alter your mind and find mental clarity.

Lift your Mood

Sometimes all it takes is a few simple actions to alter your mood. Of course, the hardest part about altering your mood is the change aspect of it. But if you give it a chance and try the ideas listed below, then you might be surprised in how much better you will feel afterwards.

- **Politeness** – Simple kindness towards others will have kindness reinforced upon you. This kindness can be as simple as saying "thank you" to your waitress or somebody who does something for you. Not only will it make that person feel good, but it will make you feel good as well.

- **Stay Offline** – People have become greatly addicted to the internet, particularly social media websites. This is a very bad habit to get into because you spend hours looking at other people's pictures and reading comments about their lives.

What are these things doing for your life? That is what you should be concerned with. Therefore, stay away from the internet for a while and replace that time with something you can do in real life. Perhaps you could exercise, read a book or hang out with a friend.

- **Getaway Plan** – We all need to get away from our daily lives and see a new environment. Even if you cannot afford to drive cross country or fly to a foreign country, you should still plan some kind of trip to get away from your town for a while.

Planning a trip is exciting because it involves adventure and travel. These are things you can look forward to as you plan your getaway. Then once you finally complete the trip, you will have memories that you can look back upon with glee.

- **Build Relationships** – Building relationships is very important in life. It can change the way you think and feel about the world in general. If your relationships are positive ones then you will feel good about the world. This will make you a happy minded person.

Whether you have lots of friends or just one, all you need is someone who you can talk to and who will cheer you up. You will be amazed how much of a difference this will make towards your attitude in general.

- **Get Sleep** – This book has already talked about the importance of sleep and how it can put you in a better mood. Sleep not only helps you physically, but it helps you focus and think better as well. Then you won't lag behind at work or in school.

  If you don't have 8 consecutive hours to sleep, then try breaking up your sleep throughout the day. There is nothing wrong with taking a nap because a few extra hours of sleep is certainly better than no extra hours.

  So next time you feel tired and stressed out in the middle of the day, set aside a few hours of snooze time. Then when you wake up, you should feel as good as new.

- **Stop Comparing Yourself to Others** – We all have our own journey in life. If you start wishing you had someone else's life by living vicariously through them, then you are going to be really unhappy when you have to go back and face your own life again.

  Instead of wishing you could do the things that other people can do, go out and learn how to do them. But don't try to do the same things as other people just because they had success with them. You have to find out on your own what makes you successful, which could be something different entirely.

Learn to focus on your own path in life. This is the most important part of mental clarity. After all, the only way you can advance is if you watch what you are doing, not what others are doing. So remember this and exceed in your own life's goals

Stress Buster 15

Slow Down

We all have memories inside our brains. These memories consist of the events that happened to us in our lives. Some of these memories are good while others are bad.

Believe it or not, people often feel stress just because they think about terrible memories of the past. As they think about these memories, they may even feel the same emotional pain they felt back then.

Memories typically come to us at random if we are not trying to think about them. We may see or hear something that reminds us of something else that happened in the past. Then we will drift off into our memories and practically start reliving them in our head.

People also get stressed out by thinking of the future and trying to imagine what their life is going to be like then. More often than not, people typically try to imagine themselves in a glorious life. This could be dreams of wealth, sex, love or power.

With such high expectations about the future, people tend to stress themselves over trying to figure out how they will make their future lifestyle a reality in the present. This just keeps generating endless amounts of stress because people will never stop imagining a better future no matter what their current situation in life actually is.

Between memories of the past and living in your dreams of the future, all of this will ultimately make you angry and create excessive amounts of stress.

Stay in the Present

We often drift off in our minds because we want to escape the present. Perhaps, we are unhappy in our lives and want to imagine ourselves in another place.

But whether you are thinking about good memories of the past or happy memories you want to have in the future, you need to just slow down your mental drifting and stay in the present.

The present is the only thing we really have control over in our lives. Sure the actions we take now will ultimately affect our futures to some degree, but nothing about the future is certain.

All we have is what we see, smell, hear, taste and feel in the present. The best we can do is work with these things to make our life better now instead of later.

You will notice something great happening when you slow down your thinking by staying in the present. You will feel less stressed by not having to imagine yourself in the past or future. After all, it takes a lot of mental power to completely transport yourself into another time and place.

By staying in the present, you don't have to use your brain to transport yourself anywhere. You are in the present, which means you can use all of your other senses to visualize where you are. This takes a lot of pressure off the brain because it doesn't have to imagine the senses for you.

How to Stay in the Present

You may be thinking that it is tough to stay in the present when you have so many things on your mind all the time. Unfortunately, we don't have a switch in our heads to turn off memories or imaginative thoughts.

To stay in the present, we must first eliminate reminders of the past. This means you should take down any photographs on your walls, both at work and home, which show something from the past. That way you won't have a visual reminder staring you in the face.

Another way to avoid mental drifting is to stop watching television. This will put images in your head that will cause you to get dozens of different thoughts at once.

Most of these thoughts won't even pertain to your own life. Instead, they will be imaginative thoughts that will clutter your mind with junk.

You should only be thinking about things that pertain to your life and that matter to you in the present. If you have studied the chapter on meditation, then you can use this practice to further enhance your abilities to focus on the present.

For a recap, meditation is the ability to train your mind to focus on one thing and nothing else. You eliminate all other thoughts, feelings, memories and emotions. Then you just focus on the one thing that brings you happiness in the present.

Go Rural

Part of the reason we think too much is because we lead such busy lives, especially if you live in a big city. There is just so much to mentally absorb throughout your surroundings.

If you have any vacation time saved up at work or free time available, think about taking a trip to a rural environment. This is an environment that is out in the woods and away from most people.

What you could do is rent a cabin for the weekend in somewhere remote. You can stay in this cabin by yourself or you can bring someone along with you. The point is to get away from the troubles and stresses of your daily life, and focus on nature.

There is something surreal about nature. For one thing, it is the most natural environment you can ever be in. Between the trees, river streams and the fresh air outside, it all has an essence to it that can make you feel better mentally and physically.

To further enhance the experience, try meditating outside in front of a stream of water. The white noise from the stream will help clear your mind as you begin to focus on your one true thought of happiness.

Enjoy Life in the Moment

Perhaps the most important lesson you can learn from this chapter is to simply enjoy your life and everything that you currently have. Don't think about what you don't have or what you'd like to have. Just enjoy what you do have.

You would be amazed how good your life really is. Think about all the advantages you likely have when compared to others in the world. You have food, shelter, money, car, job, and the ability to travel.

As far as world standards go, you are already a first-class citizen. Just enjoy that fact and stop wishing for more than what you have. Enjoy life in the moment and have fun.

Don't forget to share your thoughts on this book by leaving a review on Amazon.com. It takes just a few seconds.

Stress Buster 16

I Don't Care

If you take a good hard look at western culture, you will see how much drama there really is. Daytime television shows, such as Jerry Springer and Maury Povich, have certainly shed light on the eccentricities of everyday Americans.

Have you ever wondered why people are so dysfunctional these days? What is it that drives them to treat each other so terribly? All of this comes from worrying about things that don't really matter. Either that or they overanalyze every situation and make a big deal out of it.

Sometimes in life it is good to just say "I don't care" when it comes to things you have done wrong or things someone else has done wrong. There is no sense in dwelling on problems that cannot be changed.

For example, if someone calls you a vulgar name and you feel offended, don't let that one vulgarity ruin the rest of your day. You also shouldn't retaliate and try to get that person back either. All this will do is just cause more conflict, which will create more tension.

Another example could be saying the wrong thing when you ask a girl out on a date, which then causes her to laugh and walk away. If you are a guy then you know it can be nerve racking to get the courage to ask a girl out in the first place. What can feel even worse is saying the wrong thing to her.

Okay, so what? You don't have to let that ruin your day. Just be glad that you had the courage to say something to her in the first place. Most guys don't even make it that far, so you can feel happy with yourself that you did.

When these minor embarrassments or frustrations occur in your life, you just have to realize that they don't matter. Did these instances change your life at all? Are you still the same person? Of course you are, so stop caring what people say.

Stay Positive

The best character trait you can ever possess is to stay positive in a bad situation. These are the types of people who smile when there is a problem or a negative situation they are faced with.

This doesn't necessarily mean they are happy. It just means they are not angry or stressed. To stay positive minded, you have to know how to tell yourself that everything is going to be okay.

Another way to stay positive is to hang around other people who have the same will for positivity as you. They will help convince you that superficial comments and situations don't matter.

Friends and family are great for reminding you that little problems don't matter. How many times have your parents said to you that everything is going to be okay, while faced with a problem?

This is the kind of positive reinforcement you need to make sure you stay on the right path of positivity.

By now, you have already learned a lot about altering your mind and filling it with the positivity of the present. Use this technique to alleviate your worries and to let go of caring about little things that don't mater.

Make an "I Don't Care" List

We are all faced with comments and criticisms every day. We also experience little things that upset us, like getting cut off in traffic or getting a flat tire. These are things that can easily be rectified.

If you feel yourself getting angry or upset over a mediocre problem, then jot that problem down on a list entitled "I Don't Care." This is going to be a list of things that you should not stress yourself out over.

Just to help you with that list, here are some things that should go on it; insults, middle finger, flat tire, laughed at, embarrassment, rejection, and internet comments. This should help get you started on your list. As you continue to go about your life and experience frustrations, you should be able to add your own unique things to that list.

This is a list that could grow for a long time. Just keep it with you wherever you go. Then anytime you feel frustrated, go back and check that list to see if your issue is on there. If it is, place a checkmark next to it.

Then periodically, you will want to check your list and see which items have the most checkmarks. This will be an indication of what really upsets you the most in life and what you have to work on in order to stay positive.

What Really Matters

If you are having trouble staying positive in your life, then you have to sit down and think about what really matters to you in life. It may even be a good idea to make a list of things that matter. Some common things that matter to most people are friends, family, job, children and good health. This is a pretty accurate list of things that matter in most people's lives.

Now when you are faced with a situation that doesn't affect any of the things you wrote on your list, then you have no reason to worry or get upset over them. The only time when stress and worry would be understandable is if harm was caused to the people you care about or if you lost your job. These are situations that you simply cannot ignore because they are going to continue to affect your life.

However, this doesn't mean you have to stay negative about these bad situations. If you do then you will keep overanalyzing the situations trying to figure out how this could happen and why.

Sometimes, things just happen and there is no explanation. All you can do is move forward and stop caring about what happened in the past, even if it was tragic. Of course, you can learn from what happened and prepare better for the future.

Stress Buster 17

Limit Your Chemical Intake

We live in a world filled with chemicals. You already know the vast amount of chemicals that exist in junk food, but how about the more basic chemicals like tobacco and alcohol?

It is amazing that with all of the education on tobacco and alcohol, people still continue to smoke cigarettes and drink alcoholic beverages on a regular basis.

What's even more amazing is that the government permits these actions, despite the fact that there are so many regulations imposed against smokers and alcohol drinkers.

We all know tobacco increases the risk of lung cancer in individuals who smoke. As for people who don't smoke, they can still be at risk of secondary smoke if they simply hang around a smoker. Then their risk of lung cancer rises without them even holding the cigarette in the first place.

As for alcohol, this is a chemical that impairs your judgment after you drink it. This makes it difficult to drive carefully or to simply make a wise decision in any given situation.

So, why do people continue to drink and smoke if they know these things are bad for their health? In a nutshell, it all boils down to stress relief.

In the beginning, people typically get into these bad habits from peer pressure. Somebody will convince you that smoking and drinking is cool to do, so you try them out. Then you notice how much better you feel afterwards, which is when the bad habit begins to form.

We all have different tolerance levels to tobacco and alcohol. For example, not everybody who drinks beer on a regular basis is going to become an alcoholic. There are some who can hold their liquor and successfully know when to quit.

There are also people who don't know when to quit. These are the people who drink to relieve the painful symptoms of stress. Tobacco and alcohol are drugs that become addictive when used improperly like this.

Your body and central nervous system will develop a dependency on the drug in order to reduce stress. But after a while, you won't actually feel the effects of the tobacco and alcohol anymore. This will cause you to consume more of these drugs to try to get that relaxed feeling back. But instead, it will just create more stress and less relief.

If all of this is not enough, the cost associated with tobacco and alcohol is quite high. Many states throughout America have a tobacco tax that they place on every pack or carton of cigarettes that are purchased.

In some states, one pack of cigarettes is now over $10 because of the tobacco tax. If you are a chain smoker who smokes 10 packs of cigarettes each week, that means you are paying $100 a week just to feed your tobacco addiction.

As for alcohol, one beer at a bar could cost you upwards of $5 or more. You simply cannot afford to keep paying such high prices for something that is doing nothing to sustain your health.

How to Quit

If you are not a chain smoker or alcoholic, you are still not benefiting from taking these drugs. However, you do have the ability to limit your tobacco and alcohol because they have not addicted you yet.

To reduce the health effects they are having on your body, try cutting back the number of cigarettes you smoke and the number of beers you drink each week. This won't completely make you healthy, but it will reduce the negative impact it has on your stress levels.

Now for those who have developed a dependency on the drugs, you will need to quit them all together. But your task to quit will not be an easy one because you can't just limit your intake. You have to actually quit all together or else you will want as much of it as you can.

Alcoholics will have it the worst. They simply won't be able to quit on their own. They will need outside support from Alcoholics Anonymous. This is a support group where alcoholics come together and share their personal stories of alcohol abuse. These stories will help serve as a reminder to other alcoholics about why it is good to stay sober.

Alcoholics who are heavily into alcohol may even have to check themselves into a treatment clinic in order to receive medical care for their alcohol problem.

Clinics are basically rehab facilities that provide a controlled environment where the alcoholics can be medically treated as they suffer through their withdrawal symptoms.

After they are finished with their rehab, the symptoms of their addiction will decrease. However, they should still attend AA meetings for the rest of their life to help them stay sober. Otherwise, a relapse back into alcoholism is likely.

Alternatives

A good way to stay off of tobacco and alcohol is to find something to replace them with. Alcoholics typically like to drink coffee when they are stressed. It provides a similar type of buzz, but without the harmful effects of alcohol.

Tobacco users generally take up exercise after they quit smoking. This book has already taught you that exercise is good for many reasons that pertain to good health. The ability to quit smoking is another reason.

As you previously learned, exercise is a natural stress reliever because endorphin chemicals in your body get released and relax the central nervous system.

So when you are feeling anxious and stressed from not having your tobacco, try performing 20 minutes of cardiovascular exercise. If you have a gym nearby then go there. Otherwise, take a jog outside until you feel more relaxed.

Don't Believe the Myths

There are myths going around about electronic cigarettes being healthy because it doesn't contain any tobacco. While it is true that e-cigarettes are tobacco free, they still contain nicotine in them.

Nicotine is one of the main ingredients in tobacco that makes it addictive and unhealthy for you. Furthermore, you will still endure the negative symptoms from nicotine such as headaches, nausea, irritability and anxiety.

Therefore, don't look for a cheat way around smoking cigarettes. You simply have to quit nicotine all together or else it won't make a difference.

Discover Scientifically-Proven "Shortcuts" & "Hacks" to Lose Weight FASTER (With Very Little Effort)

For this month only, you can get Linda's best-selling & most popular book absolutely free – *Weight Loss Secrets You NEED to Know*.

Get Your FREE Copy Here:

TopFitnessAdvice.com/Bonus

Discover scientifically-proven tips to help you lose weight faster and easier than ever before. With this book, readers were able to improve their weight loss results and fitness levels. So, it's highly recommended that you get this book, especially while it's free!

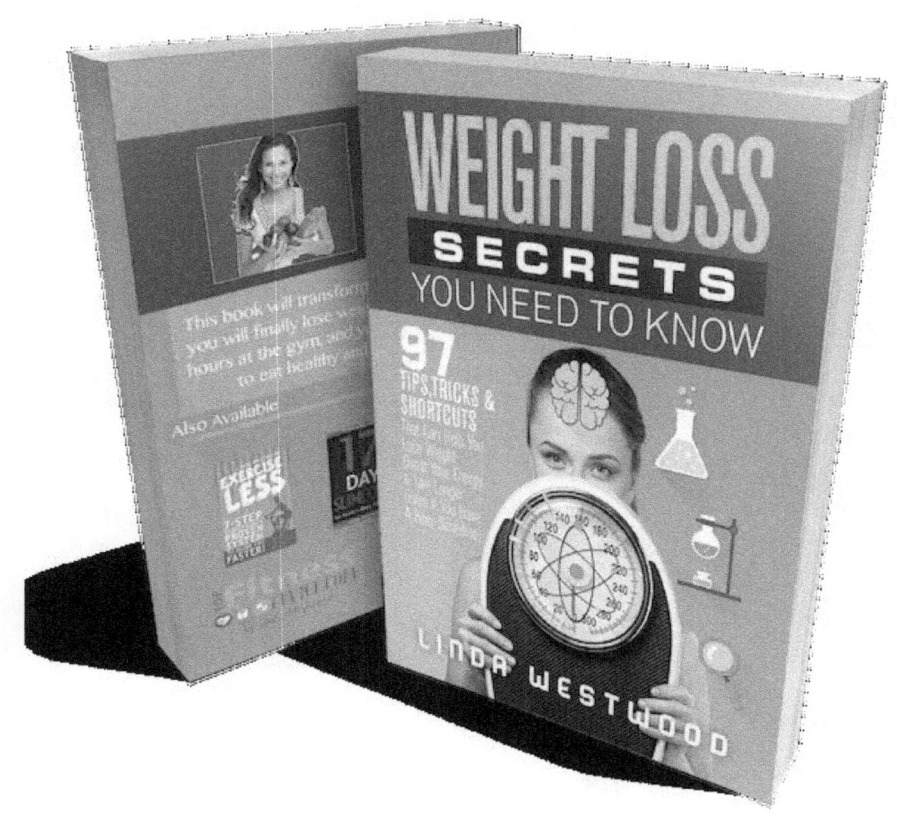

Get Your FREE Copy Here:

TopFitnessAdvice.com/Bonus

Conclusion

If you have made it this far in the book then you are clearly taking your stress management seriously. It is important for all of us to take stress seriously because it can truly have a negative impact on the quality of our lives.

There is nothing more important than health. You could be the richest person in the world who is living the perfect life, but without good health it won't even matter. You need to take care of yourself by breaking all of your bad habits and turning them into positive ones.

You should now know the differences between good habits and bad habits. The book has gone over 17 of the most common bad habits that people have and the solutions to change them into positive habits.

Did you remember to keep track of which habits in the book you currently have and don't have? How many good habits out of the 17 stress busters did you record? If the number was over 9 then you definitely aren't the most stressed out person in the world. But, you can always be less stressed so just work on the bad habits that you did record.

Now for those who recorded less than 9 good habits, you are probably on the verge of a mental breakdown. If not, then you may be in a few years if you keep going at the pace you are at. The stress must seem so unbearable that you cannot even breathe sometimes.

To successfully convert yourself away from so many bad habits, you have to take them one at a time. If you just look at all the bad habits you have and try to change them at the same time then you are going to just add on to the stress you already have.

To get started with breaking your bad habits, start with the first bad habit that you have on your list. Once you have successfully broken that bad habit, go on to the next habit on the list and so on. That way you will not feel overwhelmed by changing yourself too much at once. Nobody is that perfect.

Some bad habits might be harder to break than others. For example, you now know that social isolation is a negative habit that causes stress. But, you might initially feel so uncomfortable around other people that you don't know how to break through that and find enjoyment.

Breaking free of social isolation is a gradual process like it is when changing any bad habit. You start by hanging out with one or two people to get more familiar with not being alone.

Then when that situation becomes comfortable, you start going out to bars and parties. Eventually you will break those social barriers that keep you isolated, which will allow you to be happy again.

Do Not Give Up

The worst thing you can ever do in life is give up on your dreams of being healthier. You only have this one life to live, so if you give up on changing it for the better then you are giving up on yourself.

If you feel like you cannot change any of your bad habits then keep on trying until you do.

The world presents a lot of challenges to people. Not only that, but they inflict a lot of bad habits on them as well. If it were easy to overcome these bad habits, then you wouldn't need to read a book about how to change them. Instead, everybody would be able to change them without any hassle.

So if you ever get to a point where you feel overwhelmed with trying to change a bad habit on your list, then skip that habit for now and try to change the next habit on your list. Since some habits are easier to change than others, you want to eliminate as many habits as you can without stressing out too much.

Once you find that you have eliminated more bad habits, go back to your list and see which habits you still have left to change. You may find that you will be able to change them now because you have already eliminated so many other stressful habits from your life.

With more mental clarity, you will have the focus to make bigger changes that you couldn't make before. That is why giving up completely should never be an option. There is always a way around a problem, but it takes patience and effort.

Help Others

This book is meant to educate and inform people about how to change their lives for the better. If the information in this book helped you in your life, then you should pass on this knowledge to others.

There are billions of people in the world and not all of them have access to legitimate knowledge about changing bad habits. You don't necessarily have to recommend this book, although that would always be appreciated.

The important thing is to educate people about how their bad habits are creating stress in their lives, and that the only way to eliminate this stress is by turning bad habits into good habits. This book can always act as your guide to show them how to change these habits. Just make sure they know that there are no fancy pills or supplements that are going to alleviate stress.

Like anything worthwhile in life, you must work hard in order to achieve what you want. Stress is usually endured by people who don't try and give up on themselves all together. Since nobody can change your life for you, you have to take action.

What to Do Now

Thanks again for reading this book. If you have time, I would appreciate some feedback on the material in this book and how helpful it was to you in your life or in the lives of someone else around you.

When you are ready, I hope you find the courage to start from chapter 1 and really try to change your bad habits for the better.

Good luck and I hope you find the path to success and happiness.

Enjoying this book?

Check out my other best sellers!

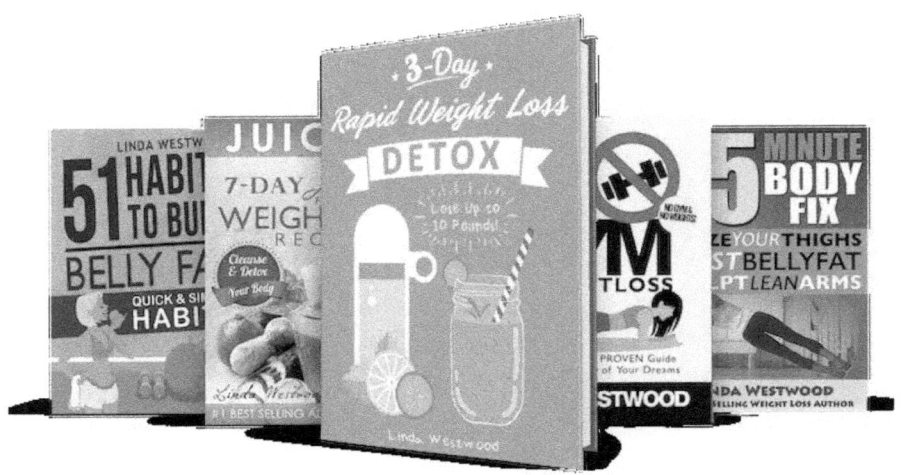

Get your next book on sale here:

TopFitnessAdvice.com/go/books

Final Words

I would like to thank you for purchasing my book and I hope I have been able to help you and educate you on something new.

If you have enjoyed this book and would like to share your positive thoughts, could you please take 30 seconds of your time to go back and give me a review on my Amazon book page.

I greatly appreciate seeing these reviews because it helps me share my hard work.

You can leave me a review on Amazon.com.

Again, thank you and I wish you all the best!

www.ingramcontent.com/pod-product-compliance
Lightning Source LLC
Chambersburg PA
CBHW031157020426
42333CB00013B/709